Sensei Self Development

Mental Health Chronicles Series

Exploring Your Identity and Self-Expression

Sensei Paul David

Copyright Page

Sensei Self Development -
Exploring Your Identity and Self-Expression,
by Sensei Paul David

Copyright © 2024

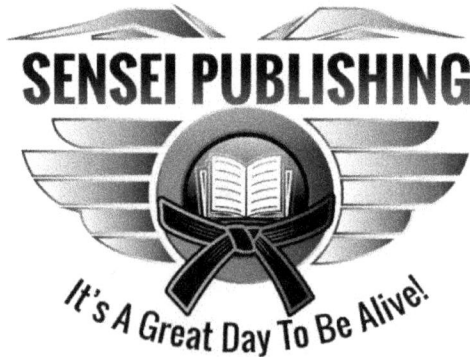

SENSEI PUBLISHING

It's A Great Day To Be Alive!

www.senseipublishing.com

@senseipublishing
#senseipublishing

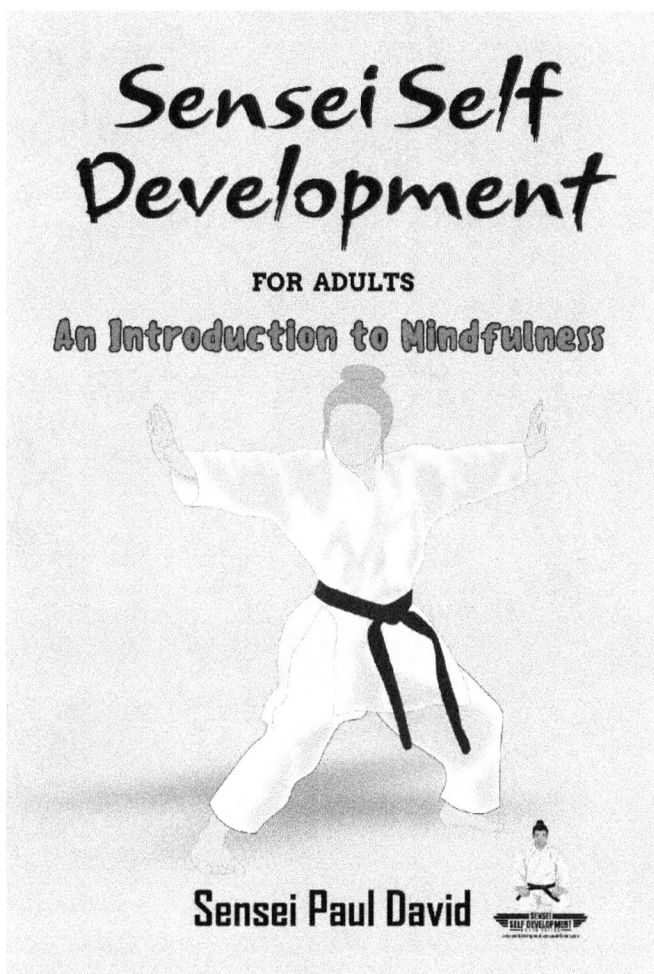

Sensei Self Development

FOR ADULTS

An Introduction to Mindfulness

Sensei Paul David

Check Out The SSD Chronicles Series CLICK HERE

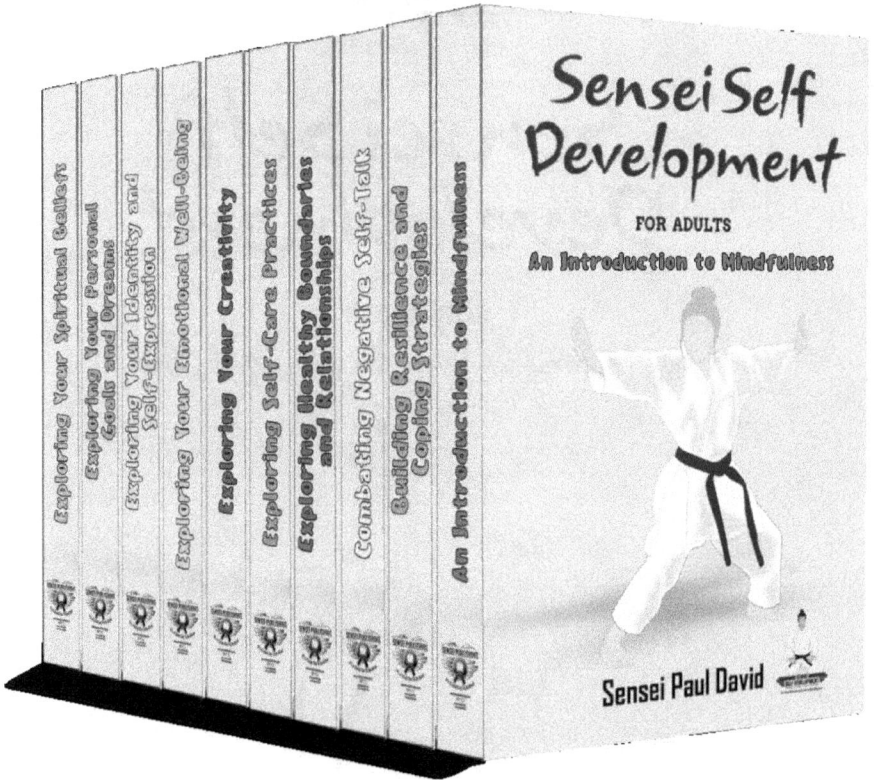

Exploring Your Spiritual Beliefs

Exploring Your Personal Goals and Dreams

Exploring Your Identity and Self-Expression

Exploring Your Emotional Well-Being

Exploring Your Creativity

Exploring Self-Care Practices

Exploring Healthy Boundaries and Relationships

Combatting Negative Self-Talk

Building Resilience and Coping Strategies

An Introduction to Mindfulness

Sensei Self Development

FOR ADULTS

An Introduction to Mindfulness

Sensei Paul David

Dedication

To those who courageously take action towards self-improvement - you are helping to evolve the world for generations to come.

- It's a great day to be alive!

If Found Please Contact:

_____

Reward If Found:

_____

MY
COMMITMENT

I, _____

commit to writing This Sensei Self
Development Journal for at least 10 days in a
row, starting: _____

Writing this journal is valuable to me because:

_____

_____

_____

_____

_____

_____

If I finish a minimum of 10 consecutive days of
writing in this journal, I will reward myself by:

_____

_____

_____

_____

_____

_____

If I don't finish 10 days of writing this journal, I will promise to:

_____

_____

_____

_____

_____

_____

I will do the following things to ensure that I write in my Sensei Self Development Journal every day:

_____

_____

_____

_____

_____

_____

Get/Share Your FREE All-Ages Mental Health eBook Now at

www.senseiselfdevelopment.com

Or CLICK HERE

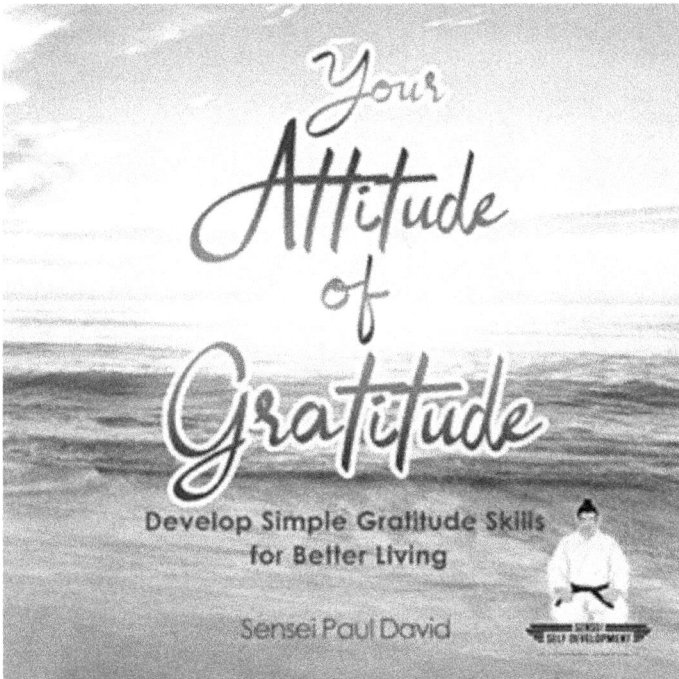

senseiselfdevelopment.com

Check Out Another Book In The SSD BOOK SERIES:

senseipublishing.com/SSD_SERIES

CLICK HERE

SENSEI
SELF DEVELOPMENT
BOOKS SERIES

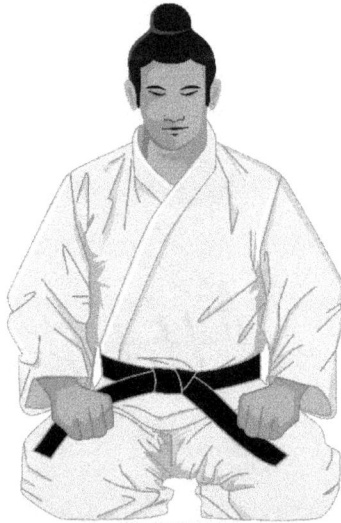

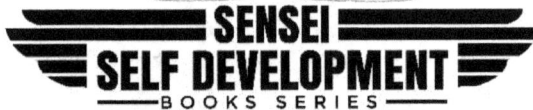

senseiselfdevelopment.senseipublishing.com

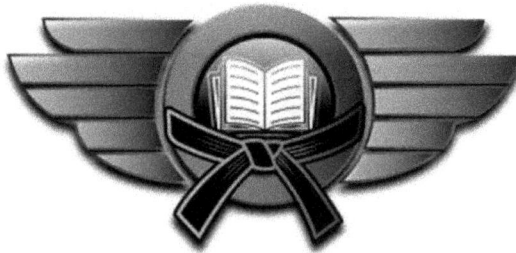

Join Our Publishing Journey!

If you would like to receive FUTURE FREE BOOKS and get to know us better, please click www.senseipublishing.com and join our newsletter by entering your email address in the pop-up box.

Follow Our Blog: senseipauldavid.ca

Follow/Like/Subscribe: Facebook, Instagram, YouTube: @senseipublishing

Scan the QR Code with your phone or tablet

to follow us on social media: Like / Subscribe / Follow

A Message From The Author:
Sensei Paul David

Dear Reader,

Welcome to the world of mental health journaling – a sacred space for self-reflection, growth, and healing. Within these pages, you hold the power to uplift your spirit, invigorate your mind, and nourish your goals.

In a world that often moves at blink-and-you'll-miss-it speed, it's crucial to make time for self-care and self-discovery.

Anxiety, stress, and emotional turbulence may have clouded your mind, making it difficult to find clarity and peace within. But fear not! Together, we will navigate the labyrinth of emotions, and experiences, helping to simplify the path to mental well-being.

This journal is not merely a bunch of blank pages awaiting your words. It is your compassionate companion, offering solace and understanding during your unique journey. Here, you are free to unburden yourself, celebrate small and large victories, and confront the challenges that may still linger.

Within the sheltered realm of these pages, there is no judgment, no expectation, and no pressure. Your unique experience and perspective hold immeasurable worth, and your voice deserves to be heard. Whether you choose to fill the lines with eloquence or simply scribble fragments of your thoughts, please remember each entry is a valuable contribution to your growth.

In this sacred space, you are challenged to take off the mask we so often wear in the outside world. It is here that you can be raw, vulnerable, and authentic – allowing your true self to be seen and embraced without reservation. By giving yourself permission to explore the depths of your emotions and confront the shadows that may lurk within, you will discover profound insights and find the healing you seek over time.

As you embark on this journaling journey, I encourage you to embrace the process itself rather than fixate solely on the outcome. Remember, it is not about reaching a certain destination or ticking off boxes on a list of accomplishments. Rather, it is about cultivating self-awareness, fostering self-compassion, and nurturing a sense of curiosity about the intricate workings of your intelligently beautiful mind.

In the quiet moments of reflection, let your pen become a bridge between your inner world and the possibilities that lie ahead. Create a sanctuary for your thoughts, fears, triumphs, and dreams. As you pour your heart onto these pages, allow your words to be a living testament to courage, resilience, and an unwavering commitment to your own well-being.

I am honored to be a part of your journey, and I believe in your ability to navigate the twists and turns with grace and resilience. Remember, you are not alone in this – countless others have walked similar paths, faced similar challenges, and emerged stronger and wiser on the other side. You have the power to reclaim all of your untapped joy, cultivate a positive mindset that serves you, and foster a deep sense of self-love and peaceful confident. – And it will take a worth effort and time.

So, open the first page of this journal with hope, curiosity, and an open heart and open mind. Embrace the transformative power of self-reflection, and allow it to guide you towards a life of greater fulfilment and peace. Each journaling session is an opportunity to not only connect with yourself but also to rekindle the light within that sometimes flickers but never extinguishes.

Remember, the pages you are about to fill are not just a record of your journey but also a testament to your strength, resilience, and indomitable spirit. Cherish this space, invest in yourself, and let your words be an ode to the magnificent journey of becoming whole.

With great respect for your decision to evolve,

Paul

MY CONVICTION

Please circle your answers below

I am DECIDING to be patient with myself and this PROCESS each time I journal toward my improved state of mental well-being

YES   NO

"The present moment is filled with joy and happiness. If you are attentive, you will see it."

Thich Nhat Hanh

Introduction

Self-expression is a fascinating and multifaceted concept that touches nearly every aspect of our lives. At its core, it's about how we convey our thoughts, feelings, experiences, and beliefs to others, and it can take many forms. From the words we choose to speak, the tone of our voice, to our body language and facial expressions, each is a method of sharing a part of ourselves with the world.

But self-expression extends beyond just our physical actions or spoken words. Art forms like painting, music, and sculpture offer more subtle yet profound ways to express ourselves. An artist can convey emotions and perspectives through their work, allowing others to glimpse their inner world.

Interestingly, while we all practice self-expression daily, it's a concept that has been somewhat sidelined in academic circles, particularly in areas like linguistics and philosophy of language. These fields have traditionally focused more on the structures of language and less on the personal, expressive aspects of communication. In social psychology, while the term self-expression is often used, it doesn't receive as much in-depth attention as one might expect given its importance in our daily lives.

Historically, self-expression was given more weight, especially in the arts and philosophy. Artists were seen as conduits for expressing deep, often unspoken, human emotions and experiences. The audience's engagement with art was viewed as a form of communion with the artist's inner world. This perspective valued the expressive power of art over its literal representation of reality.

The advent of photography and film brought about a change in this view. These technologies could capture reality in a way that painting or sculpture couldn't. As a result, the emphasis shifted from art as self-expression to art as a representation of reality. The artist was forgotten. Today, nobody talks about how a movie might reflect a screenwriter's view of the world, her likes or dislikes, and her beliefs. Only on rare occasions does that happen.

The 19th-century view of art and self-expression was closely tied to broader philosophical discussions about the nature of knowledge, emotion, and reality.

In modern times, the concept of expressiveness has been distinguished from self-expression. An artist might create a work that evokes strong emotions without those emotions necessarily being their own. This distinction has been a subject of interest in aesthetic studies.

Despite its somewhat peripheral status in academic research, self-expression remains a crucial aspect of human interaction. It's through self-expression that we share who we are with others. Whether it's through language, art, or our daily actions, these expressions are vital to human connection and understanding. They allow us to convey not just information, but also the richness of our internal lives. Understanding self-expression is key to understanding not just communication, but also the human experience itself.

Benefits of Self-Expression

Research reveals numerous benefits of self-expression. Here's a glimpse:

1. Improved Mental Health: Studies show that self-expression can lead to better mental health outcomes. Activities like writing or artistic endeavors help in processing emotions, reducing stress, and combating anxiety and depression.

2. Enhanced Self-Awareness and Personal Growth: Research indicates that self-expression aids in developing a deeper understanding of oneself.

3. Boost in Creativity and Cognitive Function: According to studies, engaging in self-expressive activities stimulates creative

thinking and enhances cognitive functions.

4. Stronger Social Bonds and Communication: Findings suggest that self-expression leads to improved communication skills and stronger relationships. It fosters empathy and understanding in interpersonal interactions.

5. Increased Confidence and Self-Efficacy: Research supports the idea that expressing oneself boosts confidence and self-efficacy, empowering individuals to voice their opinions and stand by their values.

6. Development of Emotional Resilience: Studies show that self-expression, particularly in challenging circumstances, contributes to emotional resilience, helping individuals cope better with stress and adversity.

Authentic and Inauthentic Self-Expression

When we talk about self-expression, we are always referring to authentic self-expression (since lying is technically also a form of self-expression).

Understanding the concept of the authentic self and the distinction between authentic and inauthentic expression is crucial for grasping how we interact with the world and perceive ourselves. The 'authentic self' refers to being true to one's personality, spirit, or character. It's essentially about being the real you, without pretense or suppression of your true nature. Authentic expression, then, is when your actions and words genuinely reflect this true self. Imagine saying or doing things that align perfectly with your beliefs and feelings; that's authentic expression in action. Research, like that conducted by Wood and colleagues in 2008, indicates that living authentically can lead to numerous positive outcomes, such as improved mental health and greater overall well-being.

In contrast, inauthentic expression occurs when there's a mismatch between what you say or do and what you truly think or feel. Often, this happens when people try to fit in, avoid conflict, or maintain relationships, even if it means not being entirely honest about who they are. This kind of expression, while it may serve a purpose in the short term, can lead to negative psychological effects like anxiety and depression.

The impact of inauthentic expression cannot be understated. While it might help avoid immediate problems or maintain social connections, it comes at a psychological cost. Individuals may feel compelled to express themselves inauthentically to preserve relationships, leading to mental strain. This expectation, that one wouldn't be valued for their true self, can lead to psychological distress, such as increased anxiety and depression.

Self Determination Theory and Importance of Self Expression.

Self-Determination Theory, or SDT for short, is a useful way to understand the effects of being true (authentic) or untrue (inauthentic) to ourselves. Developed by Ryan and Deci, this theory suggests that we all have three basic psychological needs: autonomy, relatedness, and competence. These needs are crucial for us to function well and feel good about our lives.

1. Autonomy: This is the need to feel in control of your own actions and life. It's about feeling that what you do aligns with who you are and your personal values.

2. Relatedness: This need focuses on our connections with other people. It's about feeling close and connected in our relationships.

3. Competence: This is the need to feel capable and effective in what we do, especially in areas that matter to us, like our work.

Now, how does SDT relate to being authentic or inauthentic?

- Authentic Expression and Autonomy: When we express ourselves authentically, it supports our need for autonomy. This is because being authentic means we are true to ourselves in our actions and words. When we can express our true selves, we feel more in control and aligned with our actions. It's like having the freedom to be who you really are.

- Authentic Expression and Relatedness: Being authentic also helps with relatedness. When we express our true selves, especially verbally, it can create stronger, more genuine connections with others. Good relationships often support and encourage us to be our true selves, fulfilling our need for relatedness.

- Authentic Expression and Competence: Finally, being able to express ourselves authentically might make us feel more competent. When we successfully communicate our true thoughts and feelings, it can boost our confidence in our abilities. This is particularly true when our actions are self-driven and not forced by external factors.

In summary, according to SDT, being true to ourselves and expressing that truth supports our basic psychological needs. It helps us feel more in control (autonomy), more connected with others (relatedness), and more capable and effective in our actions (competence). On the other hand, when we are inauthentic, we might not fully satisfy these needs, which can affect our overall well-being.

Knowing yourself + Owning yourself + Being Yourself = Authentic Self Expression

- Knowing yourself entails being aware of your personality, values, and needs. You know what you want and what you don't want.
- Owning yourself means that you can trust yourself, your opinions, thoughts, choices, and how you behave.
- Being yourself entails that you behave in accordance with your personality, values, and needs. You don't let yourself be influenced by the expectations of others.

Together, these elements lead to you expressing yourself authentically, where who you are, what you stand for, and how you behave are aligned.

How to Practise Authentic Self-Expression

Trust thyself

"Self-Reliance" by Ralph Waldo Emerson is the most impactful essay I've read. Its key message is simple: "Trust thyself." Emerson aims to embolden readers to break away from conformity and fear, nurturing the courage to listen to their own instincts.

Emerson reflects on how great artists, writers, philosophers, and prophets all disregarded traditional books and norms, choosing to express their own ideas instead. He argues that we all experience moments of profound insight, similar to those of these great minds. However, unlike them, we often overlook or suppress these insights. Emerson believes that, at some point, everyone comes to realize this truth.

"There is a time in every man's education when he arrives at the conviction that envy is ignorance; that imitation is suicide; that he must take himself for better, for worse, as his portion."

Feeling envious of great achievements means not seeing your own potential to achieve them. Copying someone else means stifling your unique qualities.

Emerson also believes that humans, God, and nature are intrinsically connected. He suggests that God communicates through us, and our moments of insight are like catching a ray of divine light. So why do we often ignore this inner divine voice? Emerson identifies two culprits: our tendencies to conform and to seek consistency.

Conformity happens when we set aside our own insights because they clash with widely accepted views. Emerson points out that traditions and popular opinions often conceal negative behaviors like racism and greed, so they alone cannot be the benchmarks of what is right.

Emerson emphasizes that we, individually, are the true judges of right and wrong, declaring, "No law can be sacred to me but that of my nature." We need to learn to overlook tradition and public opinion if they conflict with our own instincts as to what is right.

Consistency is the fear of contradicting our past words or actions. Emerson boldly dismisses this concern, stating, "A foolish consistency is the hobgoblin of little minds, adored by little statesmen and philosophers and divines. With consistency a great soul has simply nothing to do." This highlights the idea that true greatness lies in evolving beyond past selves and ideas.

Emerson argues that being overly concerned with consistency and the need to be understood limits us to trivial concerns. True greatness often requires what might look like inconsistency. Over a lifetime, these seemingly contradictory actions are like a sailboat tacking back and forth, ultimately moving in the right direction.

He suggests that it's not just the fear of being seen as odd or inconsistent that restrains us, but also an excessive respect for the past, for books, and for authority figures. The same inspiration that sparked those revered books and the inspiration we feel are identical. Elevating a ruler or king is simply recognizing the potential in any person to set their own rules. Our voices are equally valid and deserve to be heard just as much as those from the past.

Emerson acknowledges that books and individuals with superior virtue have their place. He suggests we can learn from history when we view it as a story that informs our own journey. He also speaks of a hierarchy in virtue or 'souls,' where those with greater soul influence us, and those with less are influenced by us. This, he sees as a relationship of mutual recognition and respect, rather than one of control or obedience.

Moreover, Emerson concedes that listening to our inner selves isn't the sole moral compass. We should consider our responsibilities to family, neighbors, and even pets, but ultimately, we must choose our own obligations. If societal or familial expectations push us towards certain careers or personal choices, we might be merely conforming and not following our intuition.

He illustrates self-reliance with the example of a versatile "sturdy lad from New Hampshire or Vermont," who tries his hand at various endeavors - teaching, farming, politics, real estate - without committing to a fixed career, always landing on his feet like a cat.

Emerson compares such an individual to graduates from prestigious colleges who feel like failure if they don't find immediate success, or entrepreneurs who see themselves as failures after their first business venture doesn't work out. In this comparison, the resilient and versatile "sturdy lad" is depicted more favorably. Emerson regards this type of person as being far more valuable than a hundred of these so-called "city dolls," who lack the same level of resilience and adaptability.

Know Thyself
To start living more authentically, it's also

important to know yourself better and understand what matters to you in life. This means becoming more aware of your personality, your values, and your needs.

Consider asking yourself: What do I value in my job, my relationships, and my free time? What really resonates with me? What do I enjoy, and what do I dislike? What am I good at? If I could design my ideal life, what would it look like?

These are significant questions and it's completely fine if you don't have all the answers right away, or if you're not yet familiar with this level of self-knowledge. Understanding oneself is a lifelong journey. Our wants, goals, and desires evolve over time, and their importance shifts through different life stages.

I aim to assist you in taking initial steps towards a more authentic life. There are numerous exercises that can aid in deepening your self-understanding. Let's explore some of these exercises together:

1. Visualization:

Picture it's your 80th birthday celebration, surrounded by all the people you care about. They're all eager to give a speech about you. Think about what you'd like them to say in their speeches.

Pause and ponder these questions:

1. What impact do you envision you've had on others?
2. What achievements do you hope to have accomplished by then?
3. What kind of person do you aspire to be remembered as?

What thoughts, words, or images come to mind? If possible, jot them down. The responses to these questions can reveal a lot about what you value in life.

2. Journaling

Journaling is a powerful tool for self-discovery. Establishing a daily practice of writing freely helps you tap into your subconscious. This process lets you explore your feelings, celebrate your successes, and make note of your observations. Your writing can be spontaneous, or you can use prompts for more directed exploration.

Setting aside time regularly for self-reflection is vital for getting to know yourself. To authentically express yourself involves cultivating deep self-awareness, emotional intelligence, and effective communication skills.

Cultivate Openness

To get better at self-expression, start sharing more about yourself in trusted environments. You can begin with small, less vulnerable topics and gradually move to more personal subjects as you feel comfortable.

Aim to communicate your thoughts and feelings honestly, but tactfully. Authentic expression is not just about being open, but also about being truthful in a respectful way.

Enhance Your Listening Skills:

Focus on truly hearing and understanding what others are saying. This involves not just listening to words but also paying attention to non-verbal cues like body language and tone.

Try to understand others' perspectives and feelings. This helps in forming responses that are considerate and relevant, enhancing the quality of your interactions.

Mindful Communication

Non-verbal cues can sometimes speak louder than words. Be aware of your posture, facial expressions, and gestures. Ensure they align with your verbal messages.

The words you choose can greatly impact how your message is received. Aim for clarity, avoid jargon, and be mindful of the emotional tone of your words.

Embrace Vulnerability

Acknowledge that it's okay not to have all the answers. Expressing doubts or uncertainty can be a sign of authenticity and can foster deeper connections.

When appropriate, share your struggles or failures. This can make you more relatable and approachable.

Accept Imperfection
Recognize that everyone has flaws and makes mistakes. Being hard on yourself for imperfections can hinder authentic expression.

View challenges as opportunities for growth rather than signs of inadequacy. This perspective encourages a more honest and open expression of your experiences and aspirations.

Regular Practice
Engage in discussions on a variety of topics with different people. This can help you become more comfortable in expressing yourself in diverse situations.

Consider joining a public speaking group or taking up an activity like acting or improv, which can enhance your expressiveness and confidence.

Seek Constructive Feedback
Regularly ask friends, family, or colleagues for feedback on how you express yourself. This can provide insights into areas for improvement.

If possible, seek feedback from a coach or therapist who can provide professional insights into your communication and expression styles.

Engage in Personal Development:

Professional guidance can help you understand and overcome barriers to authentic self-expression.

Attend workshops or read books on communication, emotional intelligence, and personal development. These resources can provide practical tools and strategies.

Align with Your Values

Ensure that your words and actions consistently reflect your core values. This helps in maintaining authenticity in your expressions.

Don't be afraid to express opinions that are important to you, even if they differ from the mainstream. Respectful disagreement or unique perspectives can be powerful forms of self-expression.

Remember, the journey to improved self-expression is ongoing and requires patience and persistence. Celebrate your progress along the way and continue to refine your approach as you learn more about yourself and how you interact with the world around you.

Why is Authentic Self-Expression So Hard?

Our brains are hardwired for safety. Many of us remember being singled out for being different when we were young, leading to a mindset that it's safer to just blend in. This inclination to play it safe is managed by the limbic system, a primal part of our brain that controls fight, flight, or freeze responses. It often takes a deliberate effort to go against the grain and choose being true to ourselves over conformity.

Embracing authenticity means learning to slow down. In today's fast-paced environment, we rarely take time to reflect on what we genuinely want and need. Especially in the early stages of our careers, we're so focused on establishing ourselves that we might not stop to question if this is truly our desired path. It's important to make it a practice to periodically assess how you feel about your life's direction, your goals, and what drives you.

Word of Caution

Being vulnerable and showing your true emotions is an important part of being authentic. When you're authentic, you express your inner feelings and thoughts openly, rather than hiding behind a mask. Studies show that not being able to do this can be stifling. Conforming to what others expect of us can put us in an emotional bind, leading to stress and burnout. This is especially true in high-pressure situations, like entrepreneurs pitching ideas or job interviews, where pretending to be someone you're not can make you nervous and affect your performance.

Although being fake has clear downsides, in being real, we still have choices about what parts of ourselves we reveal. There are times when it's wise to be cautious about how much we share.

In a recent study, researchers looked into how being authentic in job interviews affected the hiring chances of lawyers and teachers. They gauged authenticity by asking participants to rate their agreement with statements such as, "I try to be honest about my personality and work style when interviewing for a job," and, "It's important for an employer to see me as I see myself, even if it means acknowledging my limitations." The findings were intriguing: candidates who resonated with these statements had a higher likelihood of receiving job offers, but this was only true for those whose résumés were rated in the top 10%. For most of the lawyers and teachers, striving for authenticity didn't improve their chances. In fact, it decreased the chances for teachers in the lowest 25th percentile and lawyers in the lowest 50th percentile.

The study found that aiming for authenticity in job interviews didn't work well for most candidates and even had negative effects for some. This might be because candidates focusing on authenticity openly admitted their flaws. For applicants like lawyers and teachers with excellent résumés, this wasn't an issue;

their strengths were obvious, and admitting weaknesses showed self-awareness. However, for those who hadn't yet proven themselves, revealing their shortcomings made them appear incompetent and insecure.

In experiments, people expected to be competent were respected less when they confessed to weaknesses, like poor attention to detail, or vulnerabilities, such as seeing a therapist. This suggests that being overly authentic, without considering boundaries, can be reckless. When we share our limitations, it's important to do so without casting doubt on our strengths. This is particularly crucial for members of non-dominant groups. For example, studies show that when leaders use self-deprecating humor, men are often seen as more capable, while women are viewed as less capable. Men's competence is usually assumed, whereas women, unfairly, often have to work harder to demonstrate their competence in the workplace.

The study's findings also indicate another

reason why authenticity didn't benefit some candidates: they appeared self-centered and self-absorbed. Their emphasis on self-expression overshadowed their enthusiasm for the job and curiosity about the organization.

Herminia Ibarra, a professor of organizational behavior at London Business School, highlighted this issue on the TED podcast, WorkLife: "The problem with the 'bring your whole self to work' idea is that it can be narcissistic. What about showing interest in others?" This is supported by evidence suggesting that authenticity can be detrimental for individuals who lack concern for others. These people tend to be less liked and receive lower performance evaluations.

Authenticity, when lacking empathy, can come off as selfish. While it's important to stay true to our values, one of those values should ideally be a genuine concern for others.

So, in the end, express yourself, not always, but most of the time.

Before We Get Started…

Remember, mindfulness journaling is a personal practice, and these questions are meant to guide and inspire you. Feel free to adapt and modify them to suit your needs and preferences. Explore, reflect, and embrace the opportunity to deepen your self-awareness and cultivate a sense of inner peace.

Date ___ / ___ / ___ : S M T W Th F S

I feel:
(please circle)

because because because because because
_____ _____ _____ _____ _____
_____ _____ _____ _____ _____

Today I Am Grateful For

1. _____
2. _____
3. _____

What could help transform today into a remarkable day?

Reflective Writing

How does exploring your identity help you
understand and express yourself more honestly?

_____

_____

_____

_____

_____

_____

_____

What is the definition of self-expression?

A) The act of expressing one's thoughts and feelings
B) The demonstration of physical abilities
C) The imitation of others
D) The suppression of one's emotions

All Are Correct - Choose The Response You Feel Is Most Important To Remember

Date ___ / ___ / ___ : S   M   T   W   Th   F   S

I feel:
(please circle)

because   because   because   because   because
_____   _____   _____   _____   _____
_____   _____   _____   _____   _____

Today I Am Grateful For

1. _____
2. _____
3. _____

What could help transform today into a remarkable day?

Reflective Writing

What are the benefits and drawbacks of self-expression?

_____

_____

_____

_____

_____

_____

_____

_____

Which of the following is NOT a form of self-expression?

A) Writing
B) Dancing
C) Conforming to societal norms
D) Painting

All Are Correct - Choose The Response You Feel Is Most Important To Remember

Date ___ / ___ / ___ : S   M   T   W   Th   F   S

I feel:
(please circle)

because   because   because   because   because
_____ _____ _____ _____ _____
_____ _____ _____ _____ _____

Today I Am Grateful For

1. _____
2. _____
3. _____

What could help transform today into a remarkable day?

Reflective Writing

What is the difference between self-expression and self-exploration?

_____

_____

_____

_____

_____

_____

_____

How does self-expression contribute to identity formation?

A) It allows individuals to communicate their beliefs and values

B) It limits an individual's potential for growth

C) It creates a sense of conformity with others

D) It suppresses individuality

All Are Correct - Choose The Response You Feel Is Most Important To Remember

Date ___ / ___ / ___ : S M T W Th F S

I feel:
(please circle)

because _____ _____
because _____ _____
because _____ _____
because _____ _____
because _____ _____

Today I Am Grateful For

1. _____
2. _____
3. _____

What could help transform today into a remarkable day?

Reflective Writing

How does social media shape our sense of identity?

_____

_____

_____

_____

_____

_____

_____

What is identity?

A) A fixed set of characteristics that define a person
B) A fluid concept that evolves over time
C) A predetermined role in society
D) A set of beliefs imposed by others

All Are Correct - Choose The Response You Feel Is Most Important To Remember

Date ___/___/___: S M T W Th F S

I feel:
(please circle)

because because because because because
_____ _____ _____ _____ _____
_____ _____ _____ _____ _____

Today I Am Grateful For
1. _____
2. _____
3. _____

What could help transform today into a remarkable day?

Reflective Writing
How can you express yourself in ways that are true to who you are?

_____

_____

_____

_____

_____

_____

_____

How does self-expression differ from self-discovery?

A) Self-expression is the external manifestation of one's identity, while self-discovery is the internal exploration of one's identity

B) Self-expression is a form of communication, while self-discovery is a form of self-reflection

C) Self-expression is a conscious decision, while self-discovery is a natural process

D) Self-expression and self-discovery are interchangeable terms

All Are Correct - Choose The Response You Feel Is Most Important To Remember

Date ___ / ___ / ___ : S   M   T   W   Th   F   S

I feel:
(please circle)

because _____ because _____ because _____ because _____ because _____

Today I Am Grateful For

1. _____
2. _____
3. _____

What could help transform today into a remarkable day?

Reflective Writing

How can you use art, music, and writing to explore your identity?

_____

_____

_____

_____

_____

_____

_____

In what ways can societal expectations influence self-expression?

A) By promoting conformity and discouraging individuality

B) By encouraging free expression of oneself

C) By providing a supportive community for self-expression

D) By limiting self-expression to specific social norms

All Are Correct - Choose The Response You Feel Is Most Important To Remember

Date ___ / ___ / ___ : **S   M   T   W   Th   F   S**

I feel:
(please circle)

because _____   because _____   because _____   because _____   because _____
_____   _____   _____   _____   _____

Today I Am Grateful For

1. _____
2. _____
3. _____

What could help transform today into a remarkable day?

Reflective Writing

How does your identity shape the way you interact with others?

_____

_____

_____

_____

_____

_____

_____

How does self-expression affect relationships with others?

A) It can help build deep connections with like-minded individuals
B) It can create barriers and misunderstandings with others
C) It has no impact on relationships
D) It can make an individual more popular and socially accepted

All Are Correct - Choose The Response You Feel Is Most Important To Remember

Date ___ / ___ / ___ : S M T W Th F S

I feel:
(please circle)

:) because _____
:D because _____
:P because _____
:(because _____
>:(because _____

Today I Am Grateful For

1. _____
2. _____
3. _____

What could help transform today into a remarkable day?

Reflective Writing

What role do your beliefs and values play in exploring your identity?

_____

_____

_____

_____

_____

_____

_____

Which of the following is NOT a hindrance to self-expression?

A) Fear of judgment from others

B) Low self-esteem

C) Lack of self-awareness

D) Confidence and self-assurance

All Are Correct - Choose The Response You Feel Is Most Important To Remember

Date ___ / ___ / ___ : S M T W Th F S

I feel:
(please circle)

because because because because because
_____ _____ _____ _____ _____
_____ _____ _____ _____ _____

Today I Am Grateful For
1. _____
2. _____
3. _____

What could help transform today into a remarkable day?

Reflective Writing
How has exploring your identity changed the way
you interact with the world?

_____

_____

_____

_____

_____

_____

_____

_____

How can self-expression be a form of personal growth?

A) By allowing an individual to explore different aspects of their identity

B) By promoting conformity and limiting individuality

C) By completely suppressing one's true self

D) By encouraging stagnation and lack of growth

All Are Correct - Choose The Response You Feel Is Most Important To Remember

Date ___ / ___ / ___ : S   M   T   W   Th   F   S

I feel:
(please circle)

because _____ _____

because _____ _____

because _____ _____

because _____ _____

because _____ _____

Today I Am Grateful For

1. _____
2. _____
3. _____

What could help transform today into a remarkable day?

Reflective Writing

How have your experiences shaped the way you see yourself?

_____

_____

_____

_____

_____

_____

_____

Which of the following is NOT a factor that can shape an individual's identity?

A) Cultural background
B) Personal experiences
C) Social media influence
D) Genetics

All Are Correct - Choose The Response You Feel Is Most Important To Remember

Date ___ / ___ / ___ : S   M   T   W   Th   F   S

I feel:
(please circle)

because   because   because   because   because

_____   _____   _____   _____   _____

_____   _____   _____   _____   _____

Today I Am Grateful For

1. _____

2. _____

3. _____

What could help transform today into a remarkable day?

Reflective Writing

What are the connections between identity and culture?

_____

_____

_____

_____

_____

_____

_____

48

How does self-acceptance play a role in self-expression?

A) Self-acceptance is necessary for authentic self-expression

B) Self-acceptance limits an individual's potential for growth

C) Self-acceptance is not important for self-expression

D) Self-acceptance only affects an individual's personal beliefs and values

All Are Correct - Choose The Response You Feel Is Most Important To Remember

Date ___ / ___ / ___ : S   M   T   W   Th   F   S

I feel:
(please circle)

because _____   because _____   because _____   because _____   because _____

Today I Am Grateful For

1. _____
2. _____
3. _____

What could help transform today into a remarkable day?

Reflective Writing
How have you used self-expression to make your voice heard?

_____

_____

_____

_____

_____

_____

_____

_____

Why is it important for individuals to explore and express their identity?

A) It allows for personal growth and fulfillment
B) It is a form of rebellion against societal norms
C) It is a requirement for a successful career
D) It promotes conformity and stability in society

All Are Correct - Choose The Response You Feel Is Most Important To Remember

Date ___/___/___: S M T W Th F S

I feel:
(please circle)

because   because   because   because   because
_____   _____   _____   _____   _____
_____   _____   _____   _____   _____

Today I Am Grateful For

1. _____
2. _____
3. _____

What could help transform today into a remarkable day?

Reflective Writing
What can you do to challenge the stereotypes that shape your identity?

_____

_____

_____

_____

_____

_____

_____

_____

How can self-expression change throughout different stages of life?

A) It can become more constrained and limited as an individual gets older
B) It can remain constant throughout an individual's life
C) It can evolve and change as an individual gains new experiences and perspectives
D) It can become more conformist as an individual enters adulthood

All Are Correct - Choose The Response You Feel Is Most Important To Remember

Date ___ / ___ / ___ : **S   M   T   W   Th   F   S**

I feel:
(please circle)

because _____   because _____   because _____   because _____   because _____
_____   _____   _____   _____   _____

Today I Am Grateful For

1. _____
2. _____
3. _____

What could help transform today into a remarkable day?

Reflective Writing

How can you find ways to feel comfortable and
confident in expressing yourself?

_____

_____

_____

_____

_____

_____

_____

In what ways can social media impact self-expression?

A) It can provide a platform for individuals to express themselves freely
B) It can limit self-expression by promoting societal norms and expectations
C) It has no impact on an individual's self-expression
D) It can only influence self-expression in a negative way

All Are Correct - Choose The Response You Feel Is Most Important To Remember

Date ___ / ___ / ___ : S   M   T   W   Th   F   S

I feel:
(please circle)

because   because   because   because   because

_____   _____   _____   _____   _____

_____   _____   _____   _____   _____

Today I Am Grateful For
1. _____
2. _____
3. _____

What could help transform today into a remarkable day?

Reflective Writing
What can you do to empower yourself through exploring your identity?

_____

_____

_____

_____

_____

_____

_____

How can self-expression be a means of resistance?

A) By conforming to societal norms and expectations
B) By suppressing one's beliefs and values
C) By challenging and defying societal norms and expectations
D) By completely conforming to societal expectations

All Are Correct - Choose The Response You Feel Is Most Important To Remember

As we reach the final pages of this journey through "Positive Mindset," I want to extend my heartfelt thanks to you. Your commitment to exploring positivity and its transformative power is not only commendable but a testament to your desire for personal growth and a richer, more fulfilling life experience.

Remember, the journey towards a positive mindset is ongoing and ever-evolving. Each day presents new opportunities to apply these principles, to learn, and to grow. I encourage you to revisit these pages whenever you need a reminder of your incredible potential to foster positivity and resilience in the face of life's challenges.

As we part ways, I leave you with a quote that has been a guiding star in my journey: "The greatest discovery of any generation is that a human can alter his life by altering his attitude."

— William James.

Thank you for allowing me to be a part of your journey. May your path be filled with light, hope, and endless possibilities. Farewell, and may you carry the spirit of positivity with you, today and always.

With gratitude and best wishes,

Sensei Paul David

Reflective Writing

The End

As you close the pages of this mindfulness journal, remember that each word you've written is a step on your journey towards self-awareness and inner peace. Embrace the moments of clarity, the revelations, and even the uncertainties you've encountered along the way. Let this journal be a testament to your growth and a reminder that every day offers a new opportunity to be present, to observe, and to appreciate the simple wonders of life. Carry these lessons forward, and may your path be filled with mindful moments and serene reflections. Until we meet again in these pages, be gentle with yourself and stay anchored in the now.

Mindfulness isn't difficult, we just need to remember to do it.

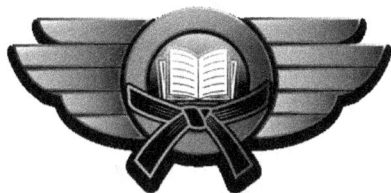

Thank You!

If you found this book helpful, I would be grateful if you would **post an honest review on Amazon** so this book can reach other supportive readers like you!

All you need to do is digitally flip to the back and leave your review. Or visit amazon.com/author/senseipauldavid click the correct book cover and click on the blue link next to the yellow stars that say, "customer reviews."

As always...
It's a great day to be alive!

Get/Share Your FREE SSD Mental Health Chronicles at
www.senseiselfdevelopment.care

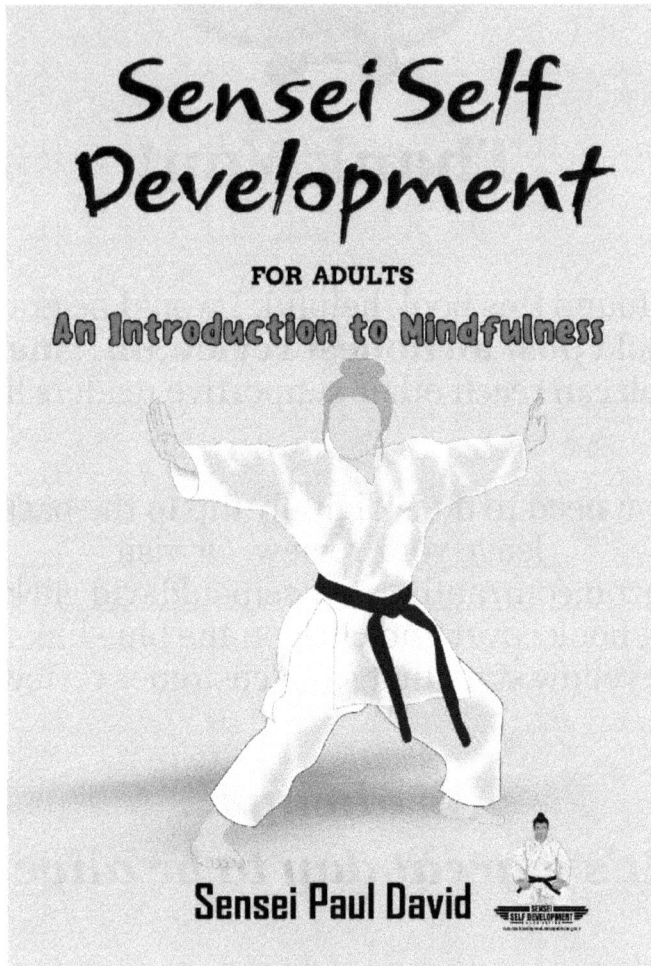

Sensei Self Development

FOR ADULTS

An Introduction to Mindfulness

Sensei Paul David

Check Out The SSD Chronicles Series CLICK HERE

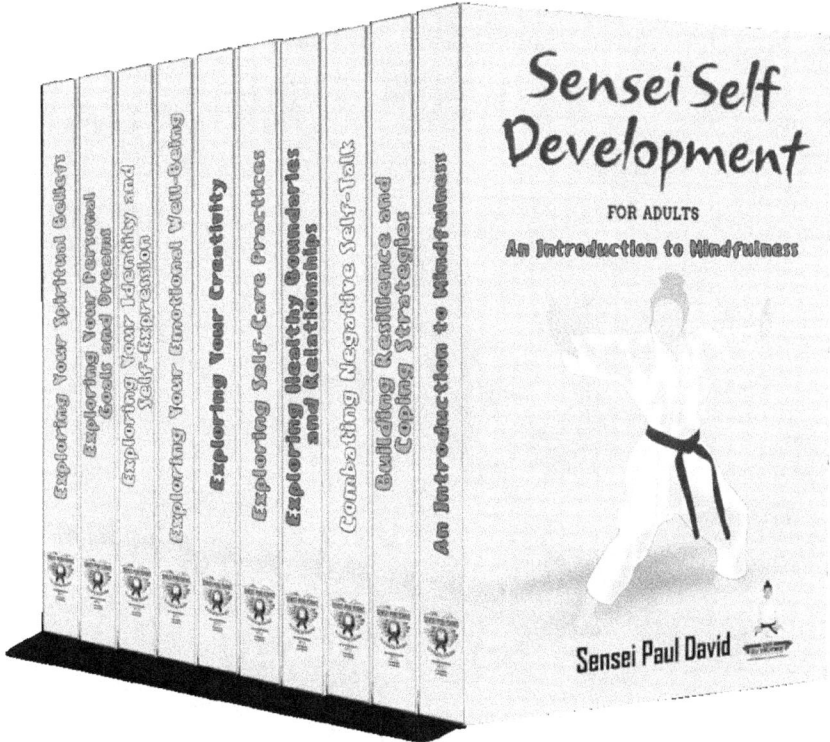

Get/Share Your FREE All-Ages Mental Health eBook Now at

www.senseiselfdevelopment.com

Or CLICK HERE

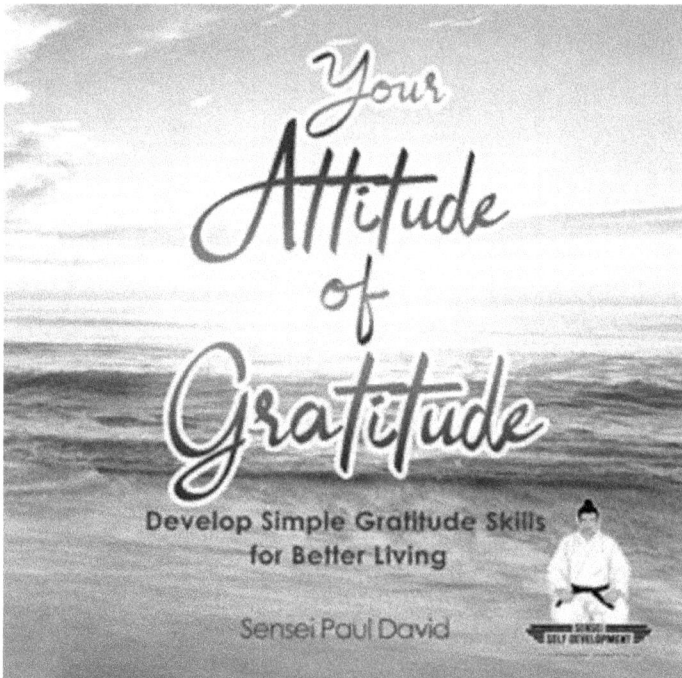

senseiselfdevelopment.com

Click Another Book In The SSD BOOK SERIES:

senseipublishing.com/SSD_SERIES

CLICK HERE

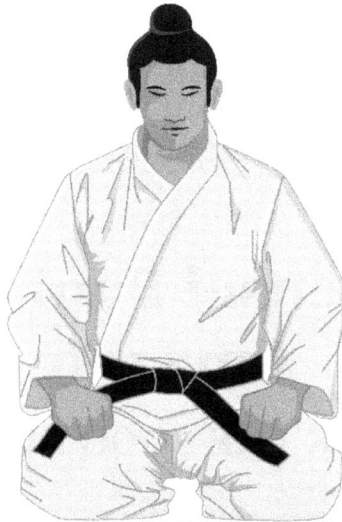

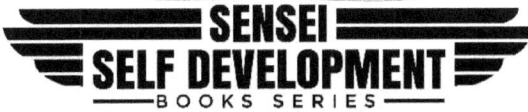

SENSEI SELF DEVELOPMENT
BOOKS SERIES
senseiselfdevelopment.senseipublishing.com

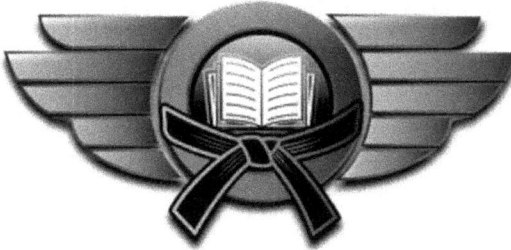

Join Our Publishing Journey!

If you would like to receive FREE BOOKS, please visit **www.senseipublishing.com**. Join our newsletter by entering your email address in the pop-up box

Follow Sensei Paul David on Amazon

CLICK THE LOGO BELOW

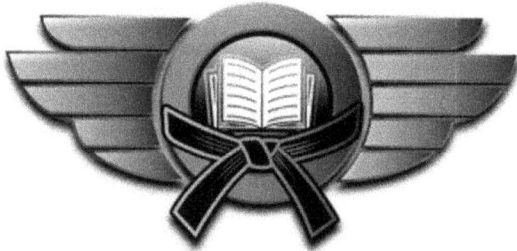

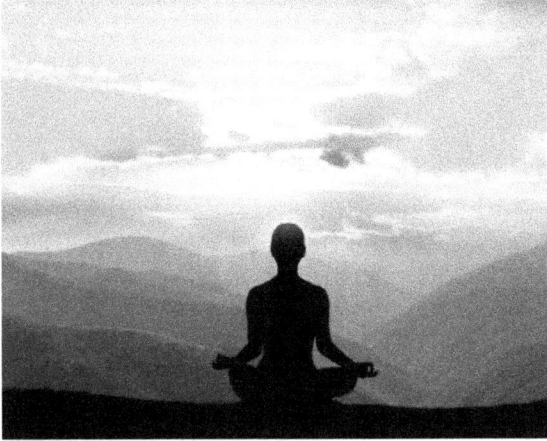

FREE BONUS!!!
Experience Over 25 FREE Engaging Guided Meditations!

Prized Skills & Practices for Adults & Kids. Help Restore Deep-Sleep, Lower Stress, Improve Posture, Navigate Uncertainty & More.

Download the Free Insight Timer App and click the link below:
http://insig.ht/sensei_paul

About Sensei Publishing

Sensei Publishing commits itself to helping people of all ages transform into better versions of themselves by providing high-quality and research-based self-development books with an emphasis on mental health and guided meditations. Sensei Publishing offers well-written e-books, audiobooks, paperbacks and online courses that simplify complicated but practical topics in line with its mission to inspire people towards positive transformation.

It's a great day to be alive!

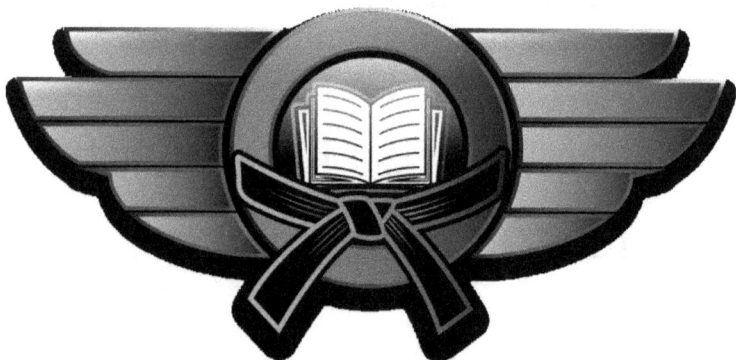

About the Author

I create simple & transformative eBooks & Guided Meditations for Adults & Children proven to help navigate uncertainty, solve niche problems & bring families closer together.

I'm a former finance project manager, private pilot, jiu-jitsu instructor, musician & former University of Toronto Fitness Trainer. I prefer a science-based approach to focus on these & other areas in my life to stay humble & hungry to evolve. I hope you enjoy my work and I'd love to hear your feedback.

- It's a great day to be alive!

Sensei Paul David

Scan & Follow/Like/Subscribe: Facebook, Instagram, YouTube: @senseipublishing

Scan using your phone/iPad camera for Social Media
Visit us at www.senseipublishing.com and sign up for our
newsletter to learn more about our exciting books and to
experience our FREE Guided Meditations for Kids & Adults.

www.ingramcontent.com/pod-product-compliance
Lightning Source LLC
Chambersburg PA
CBHW071244020426
42333CB00015B/1620